SUMMARY OF

The End Of Alzheimer's

The First Program to Prevent and Reverse Cognitive Decline

By Dale E. Bredesen, MD

Proudly
Brought To You By

OneHourReads

Copyright © 2017; By OneHourReads.
All rights reserved. No part of this publication may be reproduced, distributed, or transmitted in any form or by any means, including photocopying, recording, or other electronic or mechanical methods, without the prior written permission of the publisher, except in the case of brief quotations embodied in critical reviews and certain other noncommercial uses permitted by copyright law.

Disclaimer
This book is a summary and meant to be a great companionship to the original book or to simply help you get the gist of the original book. If you're looking for the original book, kindly go to Amazon website, and search for The End of Alzheimer's: The First Program to Prevent and Reverse Cognitive Decline by Dale Bredesen.

Table of Contents

EXECUTIVE SUMMARY 6
PART ONE: THE ALZHEIMER'S SOLUTION 8
   CHAPTER 1: DISRUPTING DEMENTIA 8
      Key Points: Alzheimer's Is Highly Feared, And For Valid Reason Too 8
      Key Points: Alzheimer's Can Be Survived 12
   CHAPTER 2: PATIENT ZERO 17
      Key Points: Alzheimer's Is Really The Result Of The Brain's Normal Functioning Gone Haywire 17
      Key Points: Terminology 20
   CHAPTER 3: HOW DOES IT FEEL TO COME BACK FROM DEMENTIA? 22
      Key Points: Recode Makes Reversal Of Cognitive Decline A Reality 22
   CHAPTER 4: HOW TO GIVE YOURSELF ALZHEIMER'S: A PRIMER 24
      Key Points: A Person's Lifestyle Patterns Determine Their Reality Of Alzheimer's 24
      Key Points: Avoiding Inflammation 25
      Key Points: Enhancing Helpful Nutrients And Hormones 27
      Key Points: Getting Rid Of Toxic Substances 28
PART TWO: DECONSTRUCTING ALZHEIMERS .. 29
   CHAPTER 5: WIT'S END: FROM BEDSIDE TO BENCH AND BACK 29

Key Points: The Scientific Unraveling Of Alzheimer's 29

Key Points: Cell Suicide Is Good For The Body, Except... 30

Key Points: Receptors Play A Fundamental Role In Triggering Alzheimer's 30

CHAPTER 6: THE GOD GENE AND THE THREE TYPES OF ALZHEIMER'S DISEASE 33

Key Points: A Person's ApoE Gene Status Is A Major Determinant Of Alzheimer's Risk Level ... 33

Key Points: Alzheimer's Disease Cannot Be Treated With A Single Drug 33

Key Points: Depending On The Triggers, Alzheimer's Disease Can Be One Of Four Types 34

PART THREE: EVALUATION AND PERSONALIZED THERAPEUTICS 36

CHAPTER 7: THE "COGNOSCOPY"- WHERE DO YOU STAND? 36

Key Points: Testing For Alzheimer's Is Never Too Early 36

Key Points: Major Markers Of Cognitive Decline And Their Optimal Levels 37

Key Points: Novel And Soon-To-Appear Tests For Cognitive Decline Assessment 43

CHAPTER 8: RECODE: REVERSING COGNITIVE DECLINE 45

Key Points: Recode Is A Targeted Program At Major Markers Of Alzheimer's 46

CHAPTER 9: SUCCESS AND THE SOCIAL NETWORK: TWO PEOPLE'S DAILY ROUTINES 49

   Key Points: Lifestyle Changes Are Necessary For The Success Of Recode 49

PART 4: MAXIMIZING SUCCESS 52

   CHAPTER 10: PUTTING IT ALL TOGETHER: YOU CAN DO IT 52

   Key Points: The Success Of Recode Depends Largely On How Early You Start, How Committed You Stay To The Program, And The Strength Of Your Support System 52

   CHAPTER 11: THIS IS NOT EASY- WORKAROUNDS AND CRUTCHES 54

   Key Points: There's A Way Around Almost Every Difficult Recode Requirement In The Course Of Treatment 54

   CHAPTER 12: RESISTANCE TO CHANGE: MACHIAVELLI MEETS FEYNMAN 56

   Key Points: Despite The Successes Recorded, A Corrupt System Stands In The Way Of Recode Getting The Acceptance And Attention Needed. 56

   Key Points: The Fight Against Alzheimers Will Benefit Greatly From A Paradigm Shift In Medical Diagnosis 57

EXECUTIVE SUMMARY

In his book, **"The End of Alzheimer's: The First Program to Prevent and Reverse Cognitive Decline",** Dale Bredesen challenges the pervading sense of hopelessness and helplessness that have trailed Alzheimer's disease. He disputes the fact that there is no effective treatment or prevention method for it, providing details of his extensive and highly successful research as evidence. His position is that Alzheimer's cannot be addressed with a single pill.

Dale dissects Alzheimer's disease, highlighting contributory factors- such as inflammation and toxic substances- that are responsible for the attendant cognitive decline in its sufferers. He explains clearly the role each plays in putting a person at risk of Alzheimer's. He also documents his highly opposed research journey culminating in the creation of ReCODE, an extensive treatment program for Alzheimer's involving components such as diet, exercise, and drugs

He describes how a person can check for each contributory factor and address the same under the ReCODE protocol. The book contains useful treatment procedures, which are also included as attached appendices.

In the book, Dave admits that, despite the recorded success and improvement in many lives, the program still has its fair share of skepticism, even from professionals who should embrace it.

Finally, he suggests ways of sustaining the impressive results recorded by the ReCODE program.

PART ONE: THE ALZHEIMER'S SOLUTION

CHAPTER 1: DISRUPTING DEMENTIA

There is no ignoring the negative perception and reality that comes along with Alzheimer's disease, from the fact that it has no known cure yet, to the fact that there's no sure way to prevent it. And this is not for lack of trying. Government organizations, neuroscientists, giant pharmaceutical companies, biotechnology experts, you name it. For decades, they have worked hard at inventing drugs, or at least finding an effective treatment. Yet, their efforts have been largely fruitless, with 99.6% of tested drugs not going beyond the testing phase. The 0.4% that do, according to the Alzheimer's association only reduce symptoms like memory loss and confusion for a limited time. Between 2000 and 2010, 244 Alzheimer's drugs were tested but only Memantine was approved by the Food and Drug Administration.

Key Points: Alzheimer's Is Highly Feared, And For Valid Reason Too

No one wants to hear a diagnosis of Alzheimer's either for themselves or for loved ones, and who can blame them? There is no positive side seen to the disease, as the name alone invokes a sense of tragedy. There are at least two reasons why we dread this disease.

For one, out of all the country's ten commonest causes of death, Alzheimer's remains the only one without a cure. Maybe with a drug to make sufferers feel a little better, we would have some form of hope. But no, there isn't. Subjective Cognitive Impairment (SCI) and Mild Cognitive Impairment (MCI), two conditions that usually manifest before Alzheimer's, have no treatment to prevent them from advancing to Alzheimer's either. It's quite unbelievable, considering all the breakthroughs that have been reached medically with other diseases in the last 20 years- cancer, HIV/Aids, cardiovascular disease, etc. If we could even hold on to some form of mushy alternate reality about Alzheimer's disease, we would. Gladly. But unfortunately, whichever way you look at it, there's just no happy ending.

The second reason there's a lot of fear about Alzheimer's is that it is beyond fatal. Before it eventually takes the life of its sufferer, it gradually tortures their very existence, robbing them of memories, putting their family and loved ones through anguish, and keeping them from living life to the fullest. Remember the 2014 movie, Still Alice, where the linguistics professor was discovered to be carrying a DNA mutation that causes its carriers to develop Alzheimer's by middle age? That discovery was made in 1995 but, unlike in other diseases where such discoveries have led to greater headway, is yet to lead to the creation of any Alzheimer's drug. It's like, with other ailments such as cancer, schizophrenia, depression, etc., progress in research continues to buoy the hope of a total cure, but with Alzheimer's nature itself seems to throw a dead end.

One minute, it's as though we're making headway, the next it's back to square one. At a time, there were results from lab studies which suggested that Alzheimer's disease develops when sticky synapse-destroying plaques are accumulated in the brain. Those plaques are created from a portion of amyloid-beta, a form of protein. The same studies suggested that amyloid-beta is formed in the brain during the course of a series of steps, and that altering those steps or destroying amyloid-beta plaques would work perfectly at preventing and treating Alzheimer's disease. Since the 1980s, most neurobiologists have upheld this hypothesis. It was so influential that the originators won various accolades for their groundbreaking work. It has also been a major deciding factor on which Alzheimer's papers get accepted for publication in top medical journals, and which Alzheimer's studies receives funding from the US National Institutes of Health.

In a sad twist, however, this amyloid-beta hypothesis did not hold true when tested in real life situations. Drug tests and clinical trials based on the rule did not only fail, in some cases, they made patients worse. Interfering with amyloid was predicted to be the almighty formula in curing Alzheimer's, but the initial studies, conducted on lab rodents, failed completely with humans.

But adherence to the ineffective amyloid theory is not the only setback to a solution for Alzheimer's. A costly assumption in medicine that Alzheimer's is a single disease, also leads to doctors treating it with donepezil (Aricept) and/or Memantine (Namenda).

Aricept works as a cholinesterase inhibitor, preventing an enzyme, cholinesterase, from destroying acetylcholine, a neurotransmitter responsible for how we think, feel, and move. Acetylcholine, which plays a huge role in memory and overall brain function, becomes reduced as a result of Alzheimer's. So with Aricept, the effect of cholinesterase is greatly reduced, allowing the Alzheimer's disease patient to remain functional for a little while longer. But this route is not without hitches. For one, it does not stop the disease from advancing. Two, it triggers the production of more cholinesterase, a fact that can pose dire consequences if for any reason the drug is stopped suddenly. Finally, Aricept comes with side effects such as headache, joint pain, nausea and vomiting, diarrhea, loss of appetite, drowsiness, and slowed heart rate.

Memantine also acts on brain chemicals to slow down symptoms of Alzheimer's disease, but only for a while. It works by preventing the transmission of brain signals from one neuron to the other following the neurotransmitter glutamate. This in turn reduces the toxic effect attached to neuronal activation. The downside to this is that it may also prevent the transmission necessary to create memories.

Bottom-line: Both drugs- Aricept and Memantine- cannot deal with the root cause of Alzheimer's or stop it from getting worse.

But beyond all these, there is a more basic problem. Alzheimer's is not just one disease, as often believed. Results from our research carried out on the biochemical differences among Alzheimer's patients indicate that there are 3 distinct classifications of the disease. Each type calls for a different treatment.

For so long, Alzheimer's disease has continued to overcome great minds in neuroscience and medicine. Obviously, we have been taking the wrong route. And if you're at risk of developing the Alzheimer's, or if you've already developed it, or have a loved one who has, it is understandable that you're very concerned. Alzheimer's disease has instilled fear in all and sundry.

Key Points: Alzheimer's Can Be Survived

However, according to the author, the disease can be prevented, and the attendant cognitive degeneration, reversed. Together with his colleagues, he trumps the norm to make certain weighty claims: that cognitive decline can be corrected, that hundreds of patients already find it possible, and that cognitive decline can be prevented, something the experts are convinced is impossible. These claims are backed by 30 years of lab research; research that successfully produced cases of first reversals of cognitive decline in early Alzheimer's disease and its signs, SCI and MCI. The author understands that their claims, as well as results from their developed therapeutic programs, may sound a little too good to be true, but asks that they keep an open mind.

This book will prove most phenomenal for people who are already in the throes of cognitive decline- be it early stage or full-blown Alzheimer's- as they will find the anti-Alzheimer's protocol life-changing indeed.

A second group, for which this book could be a life-saver, are the gene carriers. People who carry the Apolipoprotein E gene (commonly called ApoE4), are at a greater risk of developing Alzheimer's. Before now, most people preferred to stay ignorant of their ApoE status given that there was nothing to be done about Alzheimer's. Now, however, anyone can go for genetic testing, and if found to be an ApoE4 carrier, commence steps to prevent cognitive decline long before any symptoms appear.

Another group sure to benefit from this book is that of people aged 40 and above. The brain begins to age at about 40 years, and no one looks forward to a future where we'll find it difficult or impossible to carry out the basic day-to-day activities that make us who we are. Now we can lay those fears to rest, knowing that cognitive decline can be addressed, and is not irreversible as we had thought. Alzheimer's is not hopeless.

This hope, we owe to one ultimate discovery: that Alzheimer's does not occur because the brain is doing something wrong. Rather, it is as a result of one of the brain's necessary and beneficial housekeeping processes going haywire.

Although this book contains scientific evidence to support the conclusions, it is more of a practical, easy-to-use manual for the prevention and reversal of cognitive decline, as experienced in Alzheimer's or its precursors. For the 75 million Americans who carry the ApoE4 gene, the book serves as a ticket to escape the horrible fate attached to their DNA. Decades of research spun together to create ReCODE (Reversal of Cognitive Decline), a procedure that has seen many make a comeback from cognitive decline, and sustain it. ReCODE'S first patient is now 73 and has been on the program for 5 years now. She enjoys a healthy cognitive balance, which enables her to travel and work full-time.

Following the publication of this procedure in a 2014 study, thousands of emails, phone calls, and visits came in from around the world; people wanted to know more about ReCODE. And although the scientific paper contained information about ReCODE, this book provides more comprehensive and complete detail about the protocol- foods, supplements, and other useful information for anyone suffering from Alzheimer's, their physicians, and caretakers.

Adopting ReCODE holds a greater significance beyond the immediate individual. In the long run, it will take a huge load off Medicare and Medicaid, not to mention the millions of families it will free from the effects of the disease globally. There are countless testimonies, some of which you'll get to read about.

Chapters 2 to 6 explain various scientific discoveries that form the basis of ReCODE, correcting misconceptions that have long been law in the treatment of Alzheimer's.

Chapter 7 gives details about personalized tests that can reveal if you're at risk of Alzheimer's or if you already have it, and what peculiarities your condition exhibits.

Chapter 8 explains the steps to take in response to the tests. It emphasizes the fact that ReCODE is a procedure custom-fit to suit each individual's physiology, as revealed during the test.

Chapters 10 through 12 cap it off with tested tactics to sustain the results of your ReCODE procedure; helpful tips to live the best life afterwards.

Since the 19th century, conventional medicine has been built largely around diagnosis and standard 'template' treatments. But 21st century medicine continues to see more leaning towards traditional eastern approaches that make room for 'customized' medicine, so to speak. The author and his colleagues, over the course of their research, realize the need for a fusion of the best of both worlds, as this plays a major role in the prevention and treatment of Alzheimer's.

This book differs from the typical medical book in that it is built on the passion to alleviate the pain and suffering of many who have some form of experience with Alzheimer's, rather than an obligation to reel out new facts. The author does not hide that it is this passion which has seen him through every stage of research and the eventual creation of ReCODE. That passion is responsible for the breakthrough recorded in this book.

CHAPTER 2: PATIENT ZERO

Kristin was ReCODE's patient zero; the very first patient to work with ReCODE, which turned out highly successful. She had been on the verge of committing suicide after noticing symptoms which she recognized during her mother's painful battle with Alzheimer's many years earlier. The timely suggestion of a friend led her to meeting with the author and deciding to give ReCODE (at the time, an unapproved protocol) a trial. Her 'risk' paid off as she recorded massive improvements in her cognitive abilities after 3 months. Currently, she has been on the program for 5 years, suffering relapses at various times when she stopped it and regaining her abilities when she resumed it.

Key Points: Alzheimer's Is Really The Result Of The Brain's Normal Functioning Gone Haywire

At the onset of the author's research in 1989, it was widely accepted that the presence of amyloid between brain neurons is what results in Alzheimer's disease; the standard way of dealing with it was to find ways to remove the amyloid. Of course, this led to the discovery of hundreds of compounds to get rid of amyloids, with many of them producing great results in lab animals but none in patients. The situation informed the Alzheimer's Association's declaration that no drug was capable of curing Alzheimer's or halting its progress.

Kristin's results, as well as those of a few other patients who also tried ReCODE, generated a lot of interest in the protocol. It also attracted skepticism from various quarters because, apparently, it stood against existing belief about Alzheimer's; that it cannot be reversed or cured. Notwithstanding, many medical personnel have expressed interest, and been trained in this approach. More than that, physicians and neuroscientists are beginning to see Alzheimer's for what it really is- a fallout of the brain's protective function- rather than what we thought it was- an accumulation of amyloid plaques.

Basically, Alzheimer's occurs in the course of the brain protecting itself from 3 metabolic and lethal threats:

- Inflammation (from infection, diet, or other causes)
- Decline and shortage of supportive nutrients, hormones, and other brain-supporting molecules
- Toxic substances such as metals or biotoxins (poisons produced by microbes such as molds)

Chapter 6 goes into details on how these threats spark a response from the brain and how that response becomes detrimental to the brain itself. But for now, recognizing the role of these threats in the development of Alzheimer's, MCI, or SCI helps to mark out clear treatment options. First, there is need to ascertain which one or more of the 3 threats a patient's brain is responding to, after which the factors associated with the same will be removed. Those factors are responsible for initiating the accumulation of amyloid plaques, so once they're out of the way, the amyloid can be removed, followed by reconstruction of the synapses initially destroyed by the disease.

So if you do not have Alzheimer's, you can't really tell which of the 3 threats you're susceptible to. It's wise to just steer clear of any- inflammation, deficiency of supportive compounds, and/or exposure to neurotoxic materials. But if you do have Alzheimer's, SCI, or MCI already, the first step will be to identify which one or more of the threats your Alzheimer's is based on so that the best suited treatment can be administered.

This is why programmatics- a relatively new field- is employed as part of ReCODE to treat cognitive decline. It works at identifying specific contributors in individual cognitive decline cases and creates the best technique to tackle the same.

It is highly encouraged that one works towards reducing the risk of falling victim to these 3 threats. The health of our brain depends largely on how we're able to keep them away or send them packing if they're already in there. The human body is a bunch of interconnected systems, and by preventing and correcting imbalances in our biochemistry, we can prevent a disease from taking over. Keep in mind that treating your entire system might not be as quick and easy as treating a particular symptom, so brace up.

Countless factors carry the potential to aid cognitive decline. Everyone needs to know which ones they're susceptible to or which ones they're already exposed to, before a specific personalized treatment can be administered. This is what ReCODE makes possible.

Key Points: Terminology

- **Dementia-** cognitive decline that is usually heralded by memory loss and loss of the individual's mental capacity. Vascular dementia, frontotemporal dementia, Lewy body dementia, Alzheimer's, etc. are all causes of dementia. ReCODE has been proven to successfully treat Alzheimer's, SCI, and MCI, but not the other causes.
- **Vascular dementia**: a form of dementia triggered by a reduction in blood flow to the brain. It is characterized by multiple small strokes.
- **Frontotemporal dementia:** a form of dementia that causes behavioral changes, memory difficulties, and speech hitches.
- **Lewy body dementia:** this type is identified by features such as illusions, visual hallucinations, excessive sleep, etc.
- **Alzheimer's disease:** a form of dementia that is identified by the presence of amyloid plaques and neurofibrillary tangles, which can be observed with special tests. Symptoms include memory loss and severe cognitive.
- **Subjective Cognitive Impairment (SCI):** a slight decline in cognitive abilities noticeable only to the individual. With SCI, typical psychological testing will conclude the individual as normal, even though the individual can tell otherwise. After lasting for about a decade, SCI usually progresses to MCI.

- **Mild Cognitive Impairment (MCI):** in this case, neuropsychological tests reveal that something is wrong with the cognitive abilities, but the individual is still capable of carrying out certain daily activities.

CHAPTER 3: HOW DOES IT FEEL TO COME BACK FROM DEMENTIA?

Contrary to what we, as humans, generally expect of illness, Alzheimer's disease does not make you feel lousy. You have no idea something is wrong until it's quite late; when certain symptoms become impossible to ignore. Alzheimer's can progress for between 15-20 years before a diagnosis is made.

What does it feel like to descend into the abyss of dementia? Thanks to ReCODE, people who have recovered from cognitive decline can provide answers to such questions.

Key Points: Recode Makes Reversal Of Cognitive Decline A Reality

Eleanor, one of such people, began to experience symptoms of Alzheimer's at the age of 40. She faced several challenges including:

- Difficulty identifying faces and remembering names
- Feeling mentally exhausted especially in later hours of the day
- Difficulty following and participating in conversations
- Forgetfulness
- Difficulty finding the right words

Her life during this period could be described as detached from reality; she felt like there was a cloud over her brain and she watched helplessly as she lost ability to do the things she once did effortlessly.

Eleanor suffered these symptoms for nine years. Within six months of using the ReCODE program however, she noticed marked changes. And it was not just her imagination. Standard neuropsychological testing confirmed that her cognitive decline was indeed being reversed. She felt the cloud lift as she regained abilities that she had lost earlier.

- She could recognize faces and their correct names with incredible clarity
- Mental exhaustion became a thing of the past
- She could follow complex conversations easily
- She could recollect events and discussions with ease
- She no longer struggled with words or confined herself to a limited vocabulary

Eleanor's experiences are something that no one would willingly sign up for. Unfortunately, the typical American diet and way of living sets us up for just that.

CHAPTER 4: HOW TO GIVE YOURSELF ALZHEIMER'S: A PRIMER

When you consider factors that aid Alzheimer's, 3 things can happen.

- If you're yet to experience signs of cognitive decline, you get to identify those things to abstain from
- If you're already showing signs, you get to know what to cut out to reverse the cognitive decline
- You get an eye-opener of how much you're putting yourself at risk with your current lifestyle.

Key Points: A Person's Lifestyle Patterns Determine Their Reality Of Alzheimer's

Many of our daily lifestyle choices, such as eating sugary and unhealthy foods and getting insufficient sleep, put us at risk of increased insulin levels, inflammation, and damaged gastrointestinal lining. The fact that we're always busy and stressed does no good for our bodies, as it triggers the release of harmful chemicals, affecting us physically and psychologically. It doesn't help when harmful habits like smoking, are also in the mix.

It sounds pretty grim that our average day is spent heading closer to the reality of Alzheimer's. So, even though it usually takes a long time for the typical

American diet and lifestyle to take a toll, the time to nip it in the bud is now. This is what ReCODE does: initiating an all-encompassing lifestyle change that removes the threats present in each person. For the most part, ReCODE can be administered by the individual being treated. But a physician will come in handy too, for the initial testing to determine which threat(s) the brain is reacting to, and a health and fitness coach to help optimize the program.

We already know that cognitive decline is as a result of 3 major threats:

- **Inflammation,**
- **Insufficient nutrients**, and
- **Toxic exposure**- that ultimately, are linked to our diets, genetic composition, and a host of other factors.

The same factors play a huge role in not just brain, but general health. Now, although these factors are many and inter-related, it is possible to identify which ones hold potential of enhancing a particular threat. In other words, we know what to do to reduce each neurothreat.

Key Points: Avoiding Inflammation

Inflammation can occur:

- When our immune systems are triggered by the presence of disease-causing pathogens (virus, bacteria, fungi, or parasites). Usually, this is a good thing, but the process also involves the

production of amyloid, and in cases where the immune systems have to keep fighting for so long, amyloid accumulates.
- When trans-fats are introduced into the body
- When the intestines are damaged, usually as a result of eating foods containing gluten, dairy, or grains.

With the first form of attack, the key to preventing and reversing cognitive decline lies in minimizing the risk of potential infections and boosting the immune system to eliminate pathogens responsible for the same. Invariably, this reduces the amount of fighting your body has to do, controlling inflammation.

Maintaining a gluten-free diet is another effective way of preventing inflammation. Avoid foods like wheat, wheat germ, semolina, couscous, soups, cereal, ice cream, French fries, flavored coffees and teas, processed cheese, etc.

Chronic inflation is also triggered by consuming a lot of sugar, in which case, insulin resistance is also a part of the problem. Naturally, our bodies are designed to accommodate very little sugar (ideally, we should be consuming less than half of the sugars contained in a 12 ounce soft drink), but because we usually take way more than is healthy, our bodies automatically go into defense mode trying to reduce its quantity. Still, glucose- a form of sugar- remains dominant in our bloodstreams, triggering our cells to produce insulin in large quantities as a way of reducing glucose levels. Extremely high insulin levels lead to our bodies developing a resistance to its effects. As it happens, that resistance increases the chances of Alzheimer's in a person. This is why ReCODE is designed to increase a person's sensitivity, and reduce resistance, to insulin.

Key Points: Enhancing Helpful Nutrients And Hormones

In addition to halting the growth and accumulation of amyloid, it is important also to fortify the brain, making it difficult for amyloid plaques to attack your synapses. One study examined the brains of people who died in their 90s with their memory intact, and scientists discovered that they also had amyloid plaques in large quantities. There are still ongoing research but 2 tentative propositions infer that

- People who live an intellectually engaging life, create an over-abundance of synapses, enough to lose some to amyloid plaques without feeling it.
- There's a biochemical mechanism that either actively neutralize the effects of amyloid invasion, or boost the synapses enough to withstand it.

Fortifying the brain's synapses require certain nutrients, hormones and trophic factors, which the ReCODE program is designed to stimulate. A deficiency of these important substances results in the brain producing amyloid, increasing chances of cognitive decline and Alzheimer's.

Key Points: Getting Rid Of Toxic Substances

Amyloid is released when toxic substances (copper, mycotoxins from molds, etc.) are introduced into the body. Its role is to keep the poison from impairing the neurons. But we know that in the treatment of cognitive decline, one of our major goals is to prevent the production of amyloid. So ReCODE is designed to locate and destroy the source of such toxins, and remove completely every trace of it in the body through a thorough detoxification process. The ultimate goal is to eliminate any reason for the brain to produce amyloid.

Judging from how extensive this process of eliminating neurothreats is, it's quite obvious that ReCODE is not a 'one-size-fits-all' pill. It is a program targeted at the specific enhancing factors of cognitive decline in each patient; no two cases are treated the same. It may cost more time and money than the pill approach, but it does produce way, way better results.

PART TWO: DECONSTRUCTING ALZHEIMERS

CHAPTER 5: WIT'S END: FROM BEDSIDE TO BENCH AND BACK

Most readers will rather skip this part because it focuses on the scientific foundations of Alzheimer's. But it is much more than just a reporting of facts. It is an explanation of over three decades of research carried out by the author and his colleagues; their inquiries into cognitive decline, and journey towards designing ReCODE. After experiencing some events, the author's interest in the brain and its workings was piqued and, against all odds, sustained, ultimately leading to the birth of ReCODE.

Key Points: The Scientific Unraveling Of Alzheimer's

He set out to discover why brain cells- in Alzheimer's cases- deteriorate, and whether it is preset or happens by chance. The significance of this is that finding the most effective treatment for the disease would depend on which it is, unplanned or programmed. If the deterioration happened as a result of unplanned event, then it would be treated by addressing the particular event. On the other hand however, if it was something that happened as a result of a scheduled process in the brain, then treatment would require studying the process and addressing each element in it.

Key Points: Cell Suicide Is Good For The Body, Except...

The initial challenge was that unlike cells that could be extracted and grown outside the human body, it was quite impossible, at the time, to extract neurons for study. Neurologists also held the belief that such a process could not be compared to the real thing in humans, and condemned its results as unreliable. But eventually, the feat was achieved. Alzheimer's-related genes were introduced to extracted brain cells and when those cells were starved of certain nutrients or introduced to toxic substances, a series of actions were triggered, leading to the cells' decline, and eventual death. It was almost like a self-destruct command was being obeyed. This self-destruct program, in its basic form, is necessary for our survival. It is the process by which unwanted cells are destroyed and replaced, but when it occurs amidst the wrong conditions- as in the case of diseases causing cognitive decline- it's another story entirely.

Key Points: Receptors Play A Fundamental Role In Triggering Alzheimer's

The process was further broken down with the discovery of a significant relationship among receptors (responsible for carrying signals to the neurons in the brain), neurotrophins (components that aid cell wellbeing), and anti-trophin. A particular type of receptor ties in with neurotrophin, becoming a life-preserving combination for the neuron. The anti-trophin, in a cruel twist, prevents that combination, causing the affected neuron to die. That anti-trophin, in the case of Alzheimer's- is amyloid-beta.

Amyloid-beta is produced from a molecule called amyloid precursor protein, otherwise known as APP. Following a process, APP, which also happens to be a dependence receptor, can be cut in 2 different ways: at one point, to create 2 pieces, or alternatively at 3 different points to create 4 pieces. The first form of cutting produces lesser pieces than the second. As such, it hinders the development of Alzheimer's while the second triggers it. ReCODE functions by reducing incidences of the second and increasing occurrence of the first.

The next enquiry was into what defines how much of either of the two APP cutting scenarios a particular brain has. The discovery revealed that when APP attracts netrin-1, another molecule, it is cut at one spot, or it can attract amyloid-beta, in which case it causes the 3-spot division. Other factors which affect this decision include estrogen and testosterone, insulin, thyroid hormone, vitamin d, among others. This realization provided the basis for ReCODE forfeiting the 'standard drug' path. The drugs are basically good at concentrating on one thing, but these discoveries so far proved that such would be effective in treating Alzheimer's, a disease with at least 36 different influencing factors.

Not all of these contributory factors have to be treated to initiate reversal of cognitive decline, but because there is no way yet to determine which is more significant in a particular patient, the best bet is to treat as many as possible until there is noticeable improvement.

The research further established that there are two sides to making and keeping memories. One side aids the retention, and the other, loss of memories. So Alzheimer's patients have been shifted to the side supporting memory loss. Later on, Tropisetron was discovered as a drug that could shift patients from the loss side to the retention side. But Tropisetron could only address 4 out of the 36 factors, so it was suggested, as part of a clinical trial, to be used in combination with an earlier version of ReCODE. The trial, however, was met with criticism and rejection from all possible quarters. Eventually, someone- patient zero- came forward, and became the first of many. The successes recorded by these trials proved the efficacy of the program in reversing cognitive decline, SCI, and MCI.

CHAPTER 6: THE GOD GENE AND THE THREE TYPES OF ALZHEIMER'S DISEASE

Key Points: A Person's ApoE Gene Status Is A Major Determinant Of Alzheimer's Risk Level

ApoE4 is the major genetic indication that a person is highly susceptible to Alzheimer's, but how does it feature in all the research discoveries so far? APP, as was explained earlier, can be cut in 2 ways, which results in either two molecules that prevent Alzheimer's or four that support it. ApoE4 gains strength as often as the app produces the 'group of 4'. Not only does the ApoE4 encourage the retention of harmful amyloid-beta, it also attaches to the DNA, affecting up to 1700 genes in an individual.

Key Points: Alzheimer's Disease Cannot Be Treated With A Single Drug

Ultimately, these new insights into the Alzheimer's disease provide a strong basis for the most effective treatment pathway. Contrary to what most drug companies invest heavily on, Alzheimer's cannot be treated with a single drug targeting the reduction of amyloid-beta. Rather, a comprehensive program aimed at recognizing the triggers of amyloid production and reducing their chances. ReCODE does the latter, but first, it identifies which of the three types of Alzheimer's disease- *hot or inflammatory; cold or atrophic; vile or toxic-* an individual has or is at risk of.

Key Points: Depending On The Triggers, Alzheimer's Disease Can Be One Of Four Types

The Inflammatory- or Type 1- experienced mostly by people who carry one or two ApoE4 variants, is mostly hereditary and exists as a result of DNA mutations about seven million years ago. If a person inherits the ApoE4 gene from both parents, there is a very high chance of such developing Alzheimer's. Depending on how much of ApoE4 is present, symptoms can begin to appear in an individual between the forties and seventies. At the initial stage, it begins with sudden inability to retain new information. Other indications include insulin resistance and an increase in certain proteins such as tumor necrosis factor. Of all the types, this one responds to ReCODE quickly the most.

The Atrophic/Cold- Type 2- is similar to Type 1 in some ways, the only difference being that it usually displays symptoms about a decade later than the inflammatory type. It is also commonly found among people who carry one or two ApoE4 variants, and like Type 1, begins with sudden inability to recollect new information whilst retaining the ability to write, speak, and calculate. Some of its characteristics include a reduction in vitamin d and insulin resistance. The response to ReCODE is slower than in Type 1.

Between these 2 types, there is a middle, typically called type 1.5 or Glycotoxic /Sweet. Its major distinguishing feature is that glucose levels are dangerously high.

Type 3 is more common among people who carry the ApoE3 rather than the ApoE4. In other words, it is not hereditary. However, it is the most dangerous, usually following a period of extreme stress and striking early (as early as the late 40s). Symptoms usually begin with loss of cognitive abilities. Type 3 patients responded poorly to the initial version of ReCODE, prompting the intense refining of the protocol. Some of its identifying characteristics include brain damage, high level of poisonous substances in the blood, too much coper, and insufficient zinc in the blood.

The descriptions of these types explain the motivators for APP's broadcast of the four Alzheimer's-supporting pieces that are initially intended as a protective response. There's inflammation, insufficient vital nutrients (atrophic), and exposure to poisonous substances. It also depicts the different effects of amyloid-beta in each case.

Ultimately, knowledge of the types informs that an 'amyloid removal' standard approach will not work in all cases, seeing that the function in each type is different. One must test each patient for the type they're at risk of, or already suffering from, before designing the custom treatment routine that fits the same.

PART THREE: EVALUATION AND PERSONALIZED THERAPEUTICS

CHAPTER 7: THE "COGNOSCOPY"- WHERE DO YOU STAND?

Key Points: Testing For Alzheimer's Is Never Too Early

Just as most folks 50 and above are careful to get checked for cancer, there should also be efforts towards assessing one's risk level of cognitive decline factors (inflammation, insufficient nutrients, and toxicity). Whether you're out to prevent or treat cognitive decline, either way, such an assessment is necessary. And better still, it's pretty easy to get blood tests that do the job. Depending on whether a person is already showing signs of cognitive damage or at risk of the same, between 3-25 laboratory values might come up short in such tests. Such tests should be carried out early on as it becomes quite impossible to address those causes when Alzheimer's has reached the full blown state. Luckily, it usually takes a number of stages before this happens.

We have already established that these contributing factors are what should be addressed in the treatment of Alzheimer's but unfortunately, the prevailing assessment given to cognitive degeneration dangerously ignores important issues such as

- The presence and impact of the ApoE gene,
- Inflammation,
- Infections,
- Homocysteine,
- Insulin resistance
- Sufficiency, or not, of hormones
- Exposure to toxic substances like mercury and mycotoxins
- The general immune system
- The presence of bacteria
- Blood-brain barrier
- Body weight
- Prediabetes
- Volume testing for various areas of the brain

The popular methods of assessing and treating cognitive decline is one that discourages patients. Most have been told that there's no solution to the condition so they don't bother getting a medical evaluation. For others who do, they are mostly just placed on a pill or subjected to an unending series of tests.

Key Points: Major Markers Of Cognitive Decline And Their Optimal Levels

This chapter provides more insight into those 'much-talked-about' contributing factors. Here are important markers of the various factors that you should look out for:

Homocysteine

Increased levels of this amino acid is an indication of either inflammation or insufficient hormones and nutrients. It is gotten from eating foods like beef, eggs, beans, nuts, turkey, fish, dairy, shellfish, or soy.

Vitamins B_6, B_{12}, and Folate (B_9)

These are all needed in their active forms, to maintain low homocysteine. A 500-1500 pg/ml is ideal for Vitamin B_{12}, between 10 and 25 ng/ml for Folate, and 60-100 mcg/L for Vitamin B_6.

Insulin resistance

The presence of excess sugars in the body, results in a high glucose level and increased production of insulin meant to contain the glucose. Through a number of processes, these large amounts of glucose and insulin lead to the body developing an insensitivity to insulin. Extreme glucose levels can cause inflammation or insufficient brain nutrition. As such, one should stay aware of their glucose and insulin status. An ideal fasting insulin level would be 4.5 or below, while glucose should be 90 or lower.

Sugars, such as sodas and candy, as well as starchy foods like white rice, white potatoes, and white bread are foods that aid increased glucose levels.

Inflammation, Inflammaging, And Alzheimer's disease

Sometimes, the human immune system does its job a little too well. Sadly, this leads to it hurting the very body it was meant to protect, causing inflammation in the process. This inflammation, as we already know, is one of the causes of Alzheimer's. The following are indicators and measurement for inflammation:

1. High levels of c-reactive protein (0.9mg/DL is ideal)
2. Albumin-globulin ratio (at least 1.8 is an ideal measurement)
3. Omega 6-Omega 3 ratio (ideal ratio should be between 0.5 and 3)
4. Increased levels of the cytokines IL-6 and TNFα

Vitamin D$_3$

Essential for the formation and sustenance of brain synapses, a decrease in Vitamin D activity is an indication of cognitive degeneration. An ideal measurement of vitamin d3 is 50-80ng/ml

Hormonal status

Shortage of more than one hormone in the body could signal a decline in cognitive ability. They include Thyroid, Estrogens and Progesterone, Testosterone, Cortisol, Pregnenolone, and Dehydroepiandrosterone (DHEA).

Extreme copper levels and insufficient zinc

This combination is an indication and trigger for loss of cognitive function. A healthy Copper to Zinc ratio is 1:1.

Red blood cell magnesium and Ayurveda

Decreased levels of magnesium hinder optimal brain functioning. An ideal red blood cell (RBC) Magnesium level would be between 5.2 and 6.5mg/DL

Selenium the firefighter (and glutathione, the water)

Selenium works hand in hand with glutathione to rid the body of molecules that are capable of causing cognitive damage. It also works to replenish glutathione when the latter has been used up. Low selenium levels equals low glutathione levels, which can lead to cognitive damage. Ideal selenium and glutathione levels would be 110-150ng/ml and 5.0-5.5 micromolar respectively.

Heavy Metals and the Mad Hatter

Metals like mercury, lead, arsenic, and cadmium can also cause cognitive impairment. An ideal body proportion for each is below 50th percentile.

Sleepiphany: Sleep and Sleep Apnea

Inadequate sleep robs our body of metabolic processes that reduce our risk for cognitive decline. Sleep apnea is detected by an AHI (apnea-hyopnea index) evaluation. An AHI of less than 5 is okay but a perfect condition is an AHI of 0.

Cholesterol and Other Lipids

Incredibly, low cholesterol puts people more at risk of cognitive impairment than high cholesterol levels. An ideal measurement of total cholesterol for cognitive functioning in a person is more than 150.

Vitamin E

It provides protection for cell membranes and an ideal level for cognitive functioning is 12-20mcg/ml.

Vitamin B$_1$ (Thiamine)

Adequate thiamine levels improve memory formation; the ideal level of thiamine contained in red blood cells is between 100 and 150ng/ml of packed cells.

Gastrointestinal Permeability ("leaky gut")

Having a leaky gut opens one to multiple scenarios that all end in one thing: inflammation, and potentially Alzheimer's. An ideal situation is to test negative for gut permeability.

Blood-Brain Barrier Permeability

Having a leaky blood-brain barrier also opens one up to numerous pathogens that can hurt the brain. An ideal situation is to test negative for Cyrex Array 20, a blood-brain barrier evaluation.

Gluten Sensitivity and Related Sensitivities

These can lead to a leaky gut which, as discussed earlier, causes inflammation. CYREX Array 3 and Cyrex Array 4 are tests that can measure such sensitivities. The ideal condition is to test negative for both.

Autoantibodies

You need to test to see if your immune system is turning on you. Cyrex Array 5 helps provide assessment of this, and the ideal is to test negative.

Toxins, Type 3 Alzheimer's disease, and CIRS

We are constantly exposed to toxins such as molds and mycotoxins which contribute to the development of the Chronic Inflammatory Response Syndrome (CIRS) and ultimately, cognitive damage. A combination of blood tests, genetic testing, and urine sampling can be done to assess individual sensitivity to these substances.

Mitochondrial Function

Mitochondria, which provide energy for cell functioning, can be destroyed by a number of agents we regularly come in contact with. The ApoE4 gene, alcohol, antibiotics, and NSAIDS are but a few. It is possible to carry out a series of tests to assess one's status for each of the agents.

Body Mass Index (BMI)

For ideal cognitive function, a BMI of between 18 and 25 is good; visceral fat should be between 1 and 12; waistline should be less than 35 inches for females, 40 for males.

Genetics

Knowledge of your ApoE4 gene status (positive or negative) will go a long way in influencing your lifestyle choices to reduce risk of Alzheimer's.

Quantitative Neuropsychological Testing

Individual status of memory and cognitive functions can be tested to gauge one's risk level for Alzheimer's. A series of tests can be used for this, including the Montreal Cognitive Assessment (MOCA) test. A normal MOCA score is between 26 and 30.

Imaging, Cerebrospinal Fluid, and Electrophysiology

Getting a picture of our brain will reveal any problematic areas that need attention.

Key Points: Novel And Soon-To-Appear Tests For Cognitive Decline Assessment

These include Neural Extracellular Vesicles, Imaging of the Retina, and Novel Object Recognition (NOR) Test.

One area that should also be considered within the cognoscopy process is personal history and lifestyle, as this can be quite revealing in some cases.

As much as all these tests could drill a hole in the pocket of the average person, it is more economical to invest in preventing or reversing cognitive decline, than treating full-blown Alzheimer's. It is also hoped that with more ReCODE success stories, insurers will be encouraged to bear the costs of most of these tests.

CHAPTER 8: RECODE: REVERSING COGNITIVE DECLINE

ReCODE works by addressing the factors identified earlier. There are however a few points to note throughout the process:

- Treatment of each defect is aimed at restoring optimum performance.
- Treatment is geared towards not just one, but as many defects as possible
- Each treatment is aimed at the root cause of the problem a defect indicates
- ReCODE is executed based on individual defecting factors identified by lab tests
- For every treatment, there is a tipping point where the decline is either reversed or terminated
- ReCODE is an active, ongoing process. It can be modified along the way depending on individual responses.
- Drugs are only a *part* of the ReCODE program
- The earlier treatment is sought, the more chances of complete reversal there is.
- With almost every aspect of ReCODE, there's a way around the 'difficult' stuff.

Key Points: Recode Is A Targeted Program At Major Markers Of Alzheimer's

So how does ReCODE address the identified deficiencies?

Homocysteine

A combination of Vitamin B_6, B_{12}, and Folate drugs; reducing foods containing methionine, lowers homocysteine levels.

Insulin resistance

Combining the right diet with exercise (physical & mental), adequate sleep, and a stress-free lifestyle is designed to treat insulin resistance. The ideal anti-Alzheimer's diet usually administered is called Ketoflex 12/3. Aimed towards promoting ketosis and leaky gut, the diet involves a combination of Low carbohydrates, Moderate exercise, Regulated fasting, MCT oil/Olive oil, and Non-starchy vegetables.

Supplements and drugs are also administered to get optimal results.

The Promise of Sleep, Delivered

The amount of sleep a person gets eventually affects their brain function. For people who test positive for sleep apnea, the first thing to do is embark on a treatment procedure. Generally, it is advised to get as close to eight hours of sleep as possible every night without using pills. It is also necessary to cultivate the right sleeping habits. Before midnight is a good time to sleep, and the sleeping environment should be preferably dark, free from any noise and distraction.

The Surprising Effects of Stress

Stress reduction is largely based on the individual. As such, it is almost never the same for two persons. Yoga, meditation, and taking deep, slow breaths are some of the techniques applied to rid people of their stress. Reducing caffeine and alcohol intake also help.

Brain Training

Taking mental exercises, whether online or one personally developed, contributes to the improvement of cognitive ability.

Inflammation

While addressing the root cause of the inflammation, a combination of supplements (*to eliminate the inflammation*), anti-inflammatory drugs (*to prevent further inflammation*), and foods (*to eliminate root causes of inflammation*) are usually administered to patients.

Healing the Gut

First, get rid of all potential causes. Then, you can drink bone soups or use l-glutamine/colostrum capsules, or adopt the SCD diet, containing specific carbohydrates. Once the gut is sealed, probiotics and prebiotics are the next substances to absorb your diet. Finally, you should commence treatment to remove dangerous micro-organisms usually resident in the nose and sinuses.

Hormonal Balance

Optimizing hormone levels, due to controversies and challenges trailing it, is best addressed by working closely with your physician. It is highly individual-oriented as even hormonal tests only reveal the number of hormones present in a person and not the functional state.

Metal Homeostasis

High levels of mercury can be reduced by taking out your dental fillings, as well as the mercury within your system. A combination of drugs, such as zinc picolinate 25mg-50mg, and lifestyle changes, such as reduced stress, is also used to correct unhealthy copper to zinc ratios.

Toxins

Detoxification, which is quite diverse, is the major course of treatment here. It is advised that patients work with a physician in carrying out the process. One of the methods used to treat increased mercury levels is a medical procedure involving the administration of chelating agents to remove heavy metals from the body. However, there are milder alternatives that don't hurt as much. For poisoning from molds, a more complex procedure is usually applied, with the help of a specialist physician. It usually involves a combination of injections and special diet.

CHAPTER 9: SUCCESS AND THE SOCIAL NETWORK: TWO PEOPLE'S DAILY ROUTINES

Julie is one of the many success stories ReCODE has produced. She has been on the program for 5 years and has worked through so many changes. Her ReCODE journey is peculiar to her but one or two things are sure to apply to other cases.

Key Points: Lifestyle Changes Are Necessary For The Success Of Recode

Julie refused to imagine the possibility of Alzheimer's when she found out she carried two copies of the ApoE4 gene, and started showing signs of cognitive decline at 49. Not until her younger cousin developed severe Alzheimer's was she forced to seek help. Sadly, she didn't get any, but that led her to discovering ReCODE. After some months in the program, she was already showing signs of improvement.

Julie shares her daily routine which includes, among others,

GETTING ENOUGH SLEEP:

"I wake up, ideally without an alarm (not always possible) after 7 to 8 hours of sleep." (Kindle Location 3130)

EATING RIGHT:

"A typical first meal for me would be two pastured (high Omega-3) eggs with a huge plateful of colorful local, organic non-starchy vegetables. Broccoli, spinach, kale and fermented vegetables are always among my core choices. I also include a few sweet potato wedges or raw carrots for the vitamin a. I liberally use high polyphenol EVOO (Extra-Virgin Olive Oil) to finish my vegetables, along with dried sea vegetables for the iodine and pink Himalayan salt, fresh herbs and spices to season." (Kindle Location 3151)

PHYSICAL AND MENTAL EXERCISE:

"I walk or run for 50/60 minutes every single day... by challenging myself, I become stronger..." (Kindle Location 3141)

"Sometimes, I challenge myself with cognitive tasks while I walk..." (Kindle Location 3141)

AVOIDING TOXIC SUBSTANCES:

"I try to avoid any toxins in my cosmetics or toiletries..." (Kindle Location 3141)

USING SUPPLEMENTS:

"I take my evening supplements an hour or so before bed..." (Kindle Location 3183).

Julie began the program early, which improved her chances of complete reversal.

Another patient also shared her routine. In her case, she has modified the protocol to suit her, leaving out some parts yet getting tangible results. Her daily schedule is however similar to Julie's as she ticks off some major parts of the program.

SUPPORT IS VERY ESSENTIAL IN THE FIGHT AGAINST ALZHEIMER'S

The author identifies the role of social networking in global prevention of total cognitive damage. The results produced by ApoE4.info, a social networking platform created by Julie for ApoE4 carriers across the world, attest to the fact that people achieve more when they come together for a common cause.

PART 4: MAXIMIZING SUCCESS

CHAPTER 10: PUTTING IT ALL TOGETHER: YOU CAN DO IT

The totality of the ReCODE program can be expressed in 5 major areas affecting cognitive decline:

1. Inflammation
2. Insulin resistance
3. Insufficient nutrients
4. Toxins
5. Restoration and protection of missing or deteriorated synapses

Key Points: The Success Of Recode Depends Largely On How Early You Start, How Committed You Stay To The Program, And The Strength Of Your Support System

Working out the plan, however, is where most people fall short. Some of the things that have helped patients achieve success with ReCODE include:

- Starting the program as early as possible
- Adapting lifestyle to ReCODE treatment requirements
- Getting a thorough assessment of specific root causes and treating accordingly

- Continuously optimizing each aspect of the program
- Giving optimal treatment to every identified lab value
- Knowing which aspects of the program are highly necessary and which are not
- Taking note of effects following every adjustment
- Accepting that 100% reversal is not a 1-day thing
- Keeping clear records of procedures, milestones, events during the program
- Connecting with like minds, physically or online
- Avoiding sudden discontinuation of therapy

ReCODE has proven to produce greater results also in ApoE4 carriers who are yet to display signs of decline, people with SCI, early MCI, or early Alzheimer's, people who do not have type 3 Alzheimer's, people experiencing cognitive changes with no other health concerns, people with no brain atrophy, people aged below 75, and people with a strong support system.

CHAPTER 11: THIS IS NOT EASY- WORKAROUNDS AND CRUTCHES

Key Points: There's A Way Around Almost Every Difficult Recode Requirement In The Course Of Treatment

The fact that ReCODE is such an extensive program and requires many lifestyle changes, like diet, puts quite a number of people off. Some patients ignore areas they're not comfortable with, jeopardizing the procedure in the long run. But thankfully, the author identifies some alternatives for many of those unpopular areas.

- For instance, coconut milk ice-cream can be taken in place of the regular one.
- Eat organic dark chocolate in place of regular chocolate
- Satisfy sugar yearnings with MCT oil
- Quench thirst with filtered water and herbal teas
- Short on time for exercise? Try incorporating it into your daily routine.
- Finding it difficult to cut stress? Take a break. Spoil yourself with a spa day. Listen to relaxing music.
- Finding it tough to keep up with the program's many aspects? Continue monitoring your activities. Record your improvements. Soon enough, you may have no need for some parts of the program.

- Consider eating a late lunch and an early evening snack if you're having trouble keeping up with the recommended 12-16 hours fasting.

Other areas to which plausible alternatives are suggested include Meat consumption, Alcohol consumption, Smoking habits, Soy-based foods, Caffeine, Tea, Ketoflex diet, cooking with high heat, Aluminum pans, Organic food, Random cravings, and a busy lifestyle.

Overall, the strongest support throughout the ReCODE journey is the potential to rediscover oneself; evaluating previous lifestyle and finding joy in the recovery journey from cognitive decline.

CHAPTER 12: RESISTANCE TO CHANGE: MACHIAVELLI MEETS FEYNMAN

Key Points: Despite The Successes Recorded, A Corrupt System Stands In The Way Of Recode Getting The Acceptance And Attention Needed.

Often times, it is easier for people to remain skeptical about the ReCODE protocol rather than wrap their heads around it. Right from the onset of the research, skepticism and criticism have trailed the ReCODE program. From the physician suffering from early Alzheimer's disease who later experienced the effects of ReCODE and became a believer, to the G8 consultant contracted to find the solution to Alzheimer's, it has been one voice of disbelief or the other. They ranged from those who said there was no documented evidence of an effective Alzheimer's treatment, to those who thought ReCODE was just weird, or that it was too complicated for FDA approval. Unfortunately, no one was interested in how effective the program had been or how many lives and families it had improved.

Common bases for the skepticism trailing the ReCODE protocol include:

- The prevailing belief that Alzheimer's cannot be treated

- The misunderstanding that treatment is not necessary until loss of cognitive abilities set in
- The fact that none of the elements alone resemble a typical 'cure'
- Uncertainty about gluten being a contributory factor to cognitive damage
- The cost of so many required laboratory tests

And so many more.

Ultimately however, the success of ReCODE for every individual will depend on his/her determination to see it through.

Key Points: The Fight Against Alzheimers Will Benefit Greatly From A Paradigm Shift In Medical Diagnosis

Despite visible results, the ReCODE protocol will continue to receive opposition from corporate giants, myopic specialists, and their likes. Currently, there are more than one groups that have made claims of providing similar protocols to Alzheimer's patients; one group consisting of a businesswoman and a bunch of pathologists, another made up of unscrupulous it guys, both fraudulent and preying on people's desperation. Moving on, cognitive decline treatment research will have a clearer shot at success with more open minds who are not afraid of new possibilities. There must be a shift from 20th century, monotherapy-approach medicine, to 21st century holistic medicine, where each person subscribes to treatment specially designed to meet their peculiar needs. The gap between the intricacy of the human body and the present bases of diagnosis must be bridged, making it easier to accurately address chronic illnesses like Alzheimer's.

The popular belief is that no one survives Alzheimer's. This book proves otherwise.

Made in the USA
Lexington, KY
29 November 2018